Vegan Co

Building Muscle On a Vegan Diet: Vegan Recipes

By

Ralf Schmitt

Table of Contents

Introduction

Athletes prefer to adopt vegetarian diets for nutritional, economic, social, political, spiritual/religious and esthetic reasons which may include meat dislike.

While vegetarian diets are quite well-accepted in the global health arena, some coaches and practitioners raise concerns that vegetarian athletes may not get the proper nutrition needed for optimal training and success. In reality, from the various types of vegetarian foods, casual to professional vegetarian athletes can fulfil their energy and nutrient requirements. Around the same time, athletes may reduce their risk of chronic diseases and improve their ability to perform efficiently or recover from extreme exercise.

To ensure optimal efficiency, vegetarian athletes have to consume enough calories and choose foods that are rich in the nutrients of the "red flag," which are either less available in vegetarian foods or less well absorbed from plants compared to animal sources. As with most athletes, vegetarian athletes will benefit from food choices education to improve their productivity and fitness. Please read below if you want to know everything about the vegan diet and how athletes can benefit from the diet and fulfil their nutritional requirements and energy needs from plant-based foods only.

Part 1: Healthy and Delicious Vegan Recipes

Vegan recipes can often sound a little complicated and laborious. That is why below is a list of ideas for vegan breakfast, lunch and dinner that are not just tasty but quick to make. If you are just starting on a vegan diet, or trying it out for a few weeks only, or you are a plant-based expert, these 100 delicious recipes are a perfect way to figure out your weekly meal plan.

Chapter 1: Vegan Meal Prep Ideas

It takes a little expertise to recreate traditional oil-loaded classics like French fries, pesto, quesadillas, fried rice, hash browns, tacos, desserts, salads, and salad dressings without the added fat.

But do not worry: These enticing recipes use simple cooking methods such as steaming, baking, breading, pan-toasting, roasting and sautéing so you can skip the oil without skimping on flavor.

You will never run out of snacks, breakfast, lunch, dinner or dessert options with too many vegan meal planning recipes to choose from!

1.1. Smoothies and Beverages

1) Simple Strawberry Smoothie

Ingredients:

- Frozen Strawberries: 1 cup
- Soymilk: 1 cup
- Soy yoghurt: 1/2 cup
- Orange Juice: 1 Cup

Instructions:

1. Blend all ingredients, gradually adding soymilk or orange juice to reach the desired thickness.

2) Carrot, Spinach and Ginger Juice

Ingredients:

- Carrots: 4
- Spinach: A handful

- Ginger: Thumb-sized chuck

Instructions:

1. First Juice carrots, then add ginger and blend, and finally add spinach to make a delicious juice!

3) Spinach, Mango and Banana Juice

Ingredients:

- Spinach: 2 cups, freshly washed
- Chilled water: 1/2 cup
- Mango: 1 large, peeled and sliced
- Banana, 1 large, frozen (peel & freeze the banana for 2 – 4 hours before blending)

Instructions:

1. Blend the water and spinach first until liquid & frothy, then add banana and mango, and blend well until smooth.

4) Grapefruit Mango Smoothie

Ingredients:

- Mango: 1 sliced and frozen
- Grapefruit: 1 cut into slices
- Grapefruit juice: 1/2 grapefruit or whole as you like

Instructions:

1. Blend all the ingredients, gradually adding water to reach the consistency you like.

5) Mango Carrot and Banana Basil Smoothie

Ingredients

- Mango: 1, peeled and sliced
- Carrots: 2, medium-sized

- Banana: 1 frozen
- Basil leaves: 4-6 leaves
- Soy Milk: 1 1/2 Cups
- Stevia: 1 (optional)
- Ice cubes: 3-4

Instructions:

1. Blend all the ingredients until smooth.

6) Carrot Cucumber Spinach Smoothie

Ingredients:

- Carrot juice: 3/4 cup
- Cucumber juice: 3/4 cup
- Spinach juice: 3/4 cup
- Silk Vanilla: 1/2 cup
- Ice to fill up the blender

Instructions:

2. Blend all the ingredients until smooth.

7) Gazpacho Delight

Ingredients:

- Tomato juice: 2 ½ cups
- Garlic: 2 cloves
- Onion: 2 tablespoons
- Cilantro: 2 teaspoons
- Red pepper flakes: 1 half teaspoon
- Spinach: 1 tablespoon
- Cumin: 1 teaspoon

Instructions:

1. Put all the ingredients in the blender and blend until smooth.

8) Green Lemonade

Ingredients:

- Celery: 2 stalks
- Kale: 1 bushel
- Apple: 1
- Cucumber: 1 2/3
- Lemonade: 1-3 cups

Instructions:

1. Put all the ingredients in the blender and blend until smooth.

9) Carrot Mango Spinach Smoothie

Ingredients:

- Banana: 1
- Spinach: A handful
- Coconut milk: 1/4 can
- Frozen mango: 1 cup
- Baby carrots: 3
- Cinnamon: A dash or two

Instructions:

2. Blend all the ingredients, gradually adding water to reach the consistency you like.

10) Mango Carrot Cooler

Ingredients:

- Mango: 1
- Carrot: 1
- Ice cubes

Instructions:

1. Boil carrots and chopped mangos in water until the two are well cooked.

2. Let it cool and blend with ice, cumin powder, a few mint leaves, lemon juice, sugar and a little salt. Pour in a glass and serve!

1.2. Lunch and Dinner Recipes

Vegan lunch and dinner meals can either be prepared upfront and frozen in the refrigerator for up to 4 or 5 days, or assembled ahead and prepared in a slow cooker, skillet or instant oven! Preparing for certain lunches and dinners is beneficial in minimizing the tension of mealtime and saving you money (less ordering or dining out!).

1) Tofu Tacos

Made with a bit of spicy tofu filling, these fast vegan tacos make a great weekend dinner. Load them with shredded cabbage, guacamole, and fresh fresh pico de gallo to keep them vegan.

Active Time: 30 minutes | Total: 30 minutes | Servings:4

Ingredients:

- 1 tablespoon chili powder
- Ground cumin: 1 teaspoon
- Dried oregano: 1/2 teaspoon

- Salt: 1/2 teaspoon

- Ground pepper: 1/4 tablespoon

- Cinnamon ground 1/8 teaspoon

- Extra-firm tofu: 1 block (14 to 16 ounces), cut into 1/2 "cubes

- Extra virgin olive oil: 3 Tablespoons of

- Chopped onion: 1/2 cup

- Garlic cloves, minced: 2 Big

- Black beans: 1 can (15 ounces)

- Cider Vinegar: 2 Teaspoons

- Chopped cilantro: 1/2 cup

- Corn tortillas: 8 warmed

- Shredded cabbage, guacamole and pico de gallo (optional)

Directions:

1. In a medium-sized bowl, mix cumin, chili powder, salt, oregano, cinnamon, and pepper. Add and toss tofu to coat the seasonings. Rest aside

2. Add 2 tbsps. of oil in a wide non-stick skillet and put it over medium-high heat. Add onion, stir and cook for about 3 minutes until it begins to soften. Add garlic, stir and cook for 1-2 minute.

3. Raise to medium-high heat and add tofu. Cook for around 10 minutes, stirring periodically, until browning begins.

4. Add beans, stir and cook for 3-4 minutes until heated through. Turn the heat off; Stir in cilantro and vinegar.

5. To serve, add tofu filling, about 1/3 cup to each tortilla. If needed, top with the cabbage, guacamole and pico de gallo.

2) Soya Beans Hummus Wraps

This simple hummus recipe is only enough for two wraps, but the hummus is so delicious that you may want to double it and tuck it away for snacking in your fridge.

Total Prep time: 30 mins | Servings: 2

Ingredients:

- Frozen soybeans shelled (generous 1 cup), thawed: 6 Ounces
- Lemon juice: 2 Tablespoons (divided)
- Extra virgin olive oil: 2 Tablespoons (divided)
- Tahini: 1 tablespoon
- Finely chopped clove garlic: 1 tiny
- Ground cumin: 1/4 Tablespoon
- Salt: 1/4 tsp
- Ground pepper: 1/4 teaspoon of
- Green cabbage: 1 Cup, thinly sliced
- Orange bell pepper: 1/4 cup, thinly sliced
- Scallion, thin slices: 1/2
- Fresh chopped parsley: 2 Tablespoons
- Whole wheat tortilla: 2

Instructions:

1. In a food processor, mix beans, 1 tablespoon lemon juice, 1 tablespoon olive oil, tahini, garlic, cumin, 1/8 teaspoon pepper and salt. Pulse until smooth.

2. In a medium cup, whisk the remaining 1 tablespoon of lemon juice and oil with the remaining 1/8 teaspoon pepper. Add cabbage, pepper bell, scallion and parsley; stir to coat.

3. Place half of the bean hummus over each tortilla's lower third, and cover it with half of the cabbage mixture. Make a roll. Cut to serve in half, if needed.

3) Buddha Vegan Bowl

This basic bowl of grain has so many healthy ingredients: protein-packed chickpeas, sweet potatoes, creamy avocado and tahini dressing.

Active: 30 minutes | Total time: 30 minutes | Servings: 4

Ingredients:

- Sweet potato: 1 medium, cut into 1-inch pieces, peeled if desired.

- Olive oil: 3 tablespoons, divided

- Salt divided: 1/2 Teaspoon

- Ground pepper, (divided): 1/2 teaspoon

- Tahini: 2 tablespoons

- Water: 2 cups

- Lemon juice: 1 tablespoon

- Small, minced clove of garlic: 2 pieces

- Quinoa Cooked: 2 cups

- Chickpeas, rinsed, (15-ounce 1 can)

- Mature avocado, diced: 1

- New parsley or cilantro chopped: 1/4 cup

Instructions:

1. Preheat oven to 425 F.

2. Toss the sweet potato in a small bowl with 1 spoonful of oil and 1/4 teaspoon of salt and pepper. Switch to a baking sheet with rims. Bake for 16 to 18 minutes, stirring once, until tender.

3. Meanwhile, whisk each salt and pepper in a small bowl with the remaining 2 tablespoons of oil, tahini, water, lemon juice, garlic and 1/4 teaspoon remaining.

4. Divide the quinoa into 4 bowls to serve. Fill with the sweet potato, chickpea and avocado in similar amounts. Drizzle with tahini. Sprinkle with cilantro (or parsley).

4) Tijuana Torta Sandwich

A torta in the Mexican style is much like a burrito, except that the "wrapper" is a hollow-out roll, instead of a tortilla. It is loaded here with mashed black spiced beans and quick guacamole. Bring this vegetarian version to a new level (and add calcium) by rubbing the Monterey Jack cheese onto the sandwich's bean side. Serve on the cob or Spanish rice with grilled corn.

Total time: 25 minutes | Servings: 4

Ingredients:

- Black beans, or rinsed pinto beans: 1 can 15-ounce
- Salsa: 3 Spoonful
- Pickled jalapeño: 1 tablespoon
- 1/2 teaspoon of cumin
- 1 Mature avocado, pitted
- Chopped onion: 2 tablespoons
- Lime juice: 1 tablespoon

- Whole grain Baguette: 1 16- to 20-inch long
- Shredded green cabbage: 1⅓ cups

Instructions:

1. In a small bowl, mix the salsa, mash beans, cumin and jalapeno. In another small bowl, mix onion, lime juice and avocado.

2. Dice the baguette into 5 equal pieces. Cut each piece horizontally in half. Take much of the soft bread out of the middle, and you are just left with the crust.

3. Divide bean paste, avocado mixture and cabbage equally between sandwiches. Cut through and serve in half.

5) Brown Rice Bowl with Roasted Vegetables

This basic recipe of brown rice, broccoli, onions and peppers with roasted butternut squash, cashew tahini creamy sauce, and tofu marinated in lime, is a safe and fulfilling vegan lunch.

Active time: 5 minutes | Total: 5 minutes | Servings: 1

Ingredients:

- Cooked brown rice: 1/2 cup
- Roasted vegetables: 1 Cup
- Roasted tofu: 1 Cup
- Scallions sliced: 2 Tablespoons
- Fresh cilantro chopped: 2 Tablespoons
- Creamy Vegan Cashew Sauce: 2 Tablespoons

Directions:

1) Put rice, beans, and tofu in a sealable bowl or 4-cup dish. Sprinkle with the cilantro and scallions. When ready to eat, top with a sauce made with cashew.

6) **Nice Black Bean Chili and Sweet Potato**

For two, this delicious vegetarian chili is pickled with black beans and sweet potatoes. Serve with some warm corn tortillas, and toss the salad with orange and avocado segments.

Total time: 30 Minutes | Servings: 2

Ingredients:

- Extra virgin olive oil: 1 tablespoon
- Finely diced onion: 1 medium size
- Sweet potato, chopped: 1 medium size
- Garlic, minced: 2 cloves
- Chili powder: 1 tablespoon
- Cumin ground: 2 teaspoons
- Ground Chipotle, Chile: 1/4 teaspoon
- Salt: 1/8 teaspoon
- Water: 1⅓ cups
- Dry, rinsed black beans: 1 can (15-ounce)
- Diced tomatoes: 1 cup
- Lime juice: 2 teaspoons
- Fresh cilantro chopped: 2 tablespoons

Steps to prepare:

1. Using frying pan heat oil over moderate to low heat. Add onion and potato, and cook for 4-5 minutes, frequently stirring until the onion is slightly softened.

2. Add the garlic, cumin, chili powder, salt and chipotle and cook for about 30 seconds, continually stirring, until fragrant. Add water, bring to a boil, cover, rising heat to maintain a gentle boil and cook until the potato is moist and tender, for around 10 minutes.

3. Add beans, lime juice and tomatoes; raise heat to high, and return to simmer, often stirring. Reduce heat to hold a simmer and cook for around 4 minutes, until slightly reduced. Add cilantro and stir, and then remove from heat.

7) Thai Curry Noodles with Peanut

The Thai curry paste in this balanced peanut noodle recipe offers spicy kick-in-the-pants. If you have not yet tried kohlrabi, here is your excuse for buying it. The bulbous vegetable is related to the sprouts of broccoli and Brussels but has a milder, sweet taste and fabulous crunch.

Total time: 30 minutes | Servings: 4

Ingredients:

- Spaghetti of whole wheat: 8 Ounces
- Natural, smooth peanut butter: 1/2 cup
- Minced shallot: 1 small
- Curry paste Thai green, red, or yellow: 2 tablespoons
- Fresh ginger minced: 1 tablespoon
- Reduced-sodium soy sauce: 1 tablespoon
- Toasted sesame oil: 2 teaspoons

- Salt: ¼ teaspoon
- Frozen edamame: 1/2 cup, thawed
- Red peppered bell: 1 medium, cut into matchsticks
- Kohlrabi broccoli: 1 Cup, peeled, stems removed
- Fresh cilantro(optional): 1/4 cup, peeled

Directions:

1. Fill a medium saucepan of water and bring it to boil. Remove spaghetti and cook according to the instructions on the box. Reserve the liquid for 1/4 cup, then drain the spaghetti and rinse well with cold water.

2. In a big cup, whisk the reserved spaghetti water, peanut butter, shallot, curry paste, ginger, soya sauce, oil and salt. Add the rice, edamame, pepper bell, and kohlrabi (or stem broccoli); mix well to coat. If desired, serve topped with cilantro.

8) Vegetarian Lettuce Wraps

Stuff crisp lettuce leaves inspired by PF Chang's popular lettuce wraps with a savory filling. This low-carb wraps made with tofu, mushrooms and radish daikon are a simple vegetarian dinner to carry out beats! For additional snap, garnish the wraps with julienned carrots.

Prep Time: 40 minutes | Full Time: 40 minutes | Servings: 4

Ingredients:

- Rice vinegar: 3 tablespoons
- Hoisin sauce: 2 tablespoons
- Low-sodium soy sauce: 2 tablespoons
- Sesame oil: 1 teaspoon
- Crushed red potatoes: 1/4 teaspoon
- Extra-firm tofu: 1 (14 ounces)

- Canola oil: 1 tablespoon
- White mushrooms: 8 ounces, finely chopped
- Daikon radish: 1 cup finely chopped
- Garlic cloves, minced: 3 Big
- Grated ginger: 1 spoonful
- Scallions, sliced: 4
- Big Bibb or iceberg Lettuce leaves: 8 leaves
- (Optional) Julienned Carrots

Directions:

1. In a small bowl, combine vinegar, hoisin, soya sauce, sesame oil and crushed red pepper and set aside.

2. Slice the tofu horizontally in half. Remove as much water as possible, pressing the tofu slices between paper towels. Crumble it.

3. Heat the canola oil over medium to high heat in a large non-stick skillet. Add the crumbled tofu; cook, stir and break into smaller bits, about 5 minutes before you start browning.

1) Add mushrooms; continue cooking and stirring for about 3 minutes, until any liquid has evaporated.

2) Add ginger, garlic daikon and scallions. Add the reserved sauce; cook for about 2 minutes, stirring, until well mixed and heated through.

3) Spoon each lettuce leaf with a little 1/2 cup tofu mixture. When needed, top with carrots.

9) Purple Artichoke Pizza & Asparagus

Lemon and pecorino top off this tasty, easy home-made pizza which gets vibrant asparagus and artichoke color. Shiso is a mint family Fuzzy-leafed herb that is used in several Asian cuisines. It is rising in their gardens by devoted fans; look for it on Asian and farmer's markets.

Preparation Time: 24-25 Minutes | Servings: 5

Ingredients:

- Cornmeal: 1 tablespoon
- Whole-wheat pizza dough, at room temperature: 1 pound
- Extra-virgin olive oil, divided: 2 tablespoons
- Garlic sliced: 2 cloves
- kosher salt divided: ¼ teaspoon
- Crushed red pepper: ⅛ teaspoon
- Mozzarella cheese: 1½ cups shredded part-skim
- Baby purple artichokes: 2
- Lemon zest: 1 teaspoon
- Lemon juice: 2 tablespoons
- Purple asparagus: 8 ounces, trimmed
- Grated pecorino cheese: 2 ounces (1/2 cup)
- Ground pepper: ¼ teaspoon
- Purple shiso leaves (for serving)

Instructions:

1. Preheat the lower third of oven rack to 450 degrees F. Sprinkle with cornmeal over a baking sheet.

2. Roll out dough into a 12-inch oval on a lightly floured surface. Move to the prepared saucepan and brush with 1 spoonful of oil.

3. Sprinkle with garlic, 1/8 teaspoon salt and crushed red pepper, then mozzarella on top. Bake the dough for about 12 to 15 minutes, until golden brown and bubbling.

4. Meanwhile, pick off artichokes from the tough outer leaves and cut off the top two-thirds, down to the middle.

5. Peel the tough stem and remove any fuzzy choke by cutting the artichokes in half. Slice the artichokes thinly, and mix with lemon juice in a cup.

6. Using a vegetable peeler, peel asparagus into long strips; thinly slice what cannot be rasped.

7. Add the asparagus and pecorino, pepper, the remaining 1 tablespoon oil and 1/8 teaspoon salt into the bowl; mix to coat.

8. Put the vegetables on the pizza and sprinkle with zest of lemon and shiso, if required.

10) Stuffed Potatoes with Salsa Beans Salsa

With this basic recipe of loaded sweet potatoes with beans, salsa and avocados, Taco night means baked potato night. This balanced yet simple family dinner needs only 10 minutes active time so you can easily make it on the busiest weeknights too.

Active Time: 10-15 minutes | Total Time: 25-30 minutes | Servings: 4 | Calories: 324 kcal

Ingredients:

- Russet potatoes: 4 mediums
- Fresh salsa: ½ cup

- Avocado: 1, sliced

- Pinto beans: 1 can (15 ounces), boiled and lightly mashed

- Pickled jalapeños: 4 teaspoons, chopped

Directions:

1. Pierce potatoes using a fork. Microwave for 20-22 minutes, turning the sides until moist.

2. Switch to a cutting board and allow them to cool.

3. Once cool cut the potatoes in cubes using a knife.

4. Top with avocado, beans, salsa and jalapenos on each potato. Serve!

11) Rice Black Bean Bowl with Tofu and Asparagus

Black beans and sesame seeds have potent antioxidant compounds which have been proven to minimize inflammation—eating these with black rice upgrades the nutrition. Simmer it in coconut milk to add rich flavor and aroma.

Active Time: 35 minutes| Total Time: 1 hour| Servings: 4| Calories: 577 kcal

Ingredients:

- Avocado oil: 3 tablespoons, divided

- Lemongrass: 1 tablespoon, chopped

- Garlic: 3 teaspoons, minced

- Black rice: 1 cup

- Coconut milk: 1 can (15 ounces)

- Water: ⅓ cup

- Salt: ¾ teaspoon, divided

- Sesame oil: 2 tablespoons toasted

- Tamari or soy sauce: 2 tablespoons, low-sodium
- Brown sugar: 1 tablespoon
- Red pepper: ¼ teaspoon crushed
- Extra-firm tofu: 1 package (14 ounces)
- Purple asparagus: 1 pound, trimmed and cut into 1-inch pieces
- Ginger: 1 tablespoon, grated
- Shredded coconut: ½ cup, unsweetened
- Lime juice: 1 tablespoon
- Black sesame seeds: 1 teaspoon
- 3 scallions, sliced
- For garnish: Thinly sliced purple daikon and basil leaves
- For serving: lime wedges

Directions:

1. Heat 1 tablespoon of avocado oil over low-medium heat in a saucepan. Add 1 tsp of garlic and lemongrass and cook, frequently stirring for around 30-35 seconds until fragrant. Add rice and mix. Add water, coconut milk and 1/2 tsp salt.

2. Simmer over high heat. Lower heat and cook for 35-45 minutes until the rice is soft and the water is absorbed.

3. Meanwhile, take a small bowl and mix tamari, sesame oil, brown sugar and red pepper. Cut the tofu into small cubes. Use paper towels to drain excess water.

4. Heat the rest 2 tbsps. of avocado oil over medium heat in a broad skillet. Add tofu in oil and cook, tossing once, for a minimum of 8-10 minutes until crispy and golden. Transfer to a dish and sprinkle 1/4 tsp of salt over it.

5. Add ginger, asparagus, and the remainder 2 tsp of garlic to the pan; cook, stirring, for about 3-4 minutes, until the asparagus is crispy and tender. Turn off heat. Whisk the sauce, then add the tofu to the sauce.

6. Add lime and coconut juice in rice.

7. Top the tofu mixture, scallions and sesame seeds over the rice. For serving use lime wedges and, where appropriate, garnish with daikon and basil.

12) Penne Pasta with Roasted Red Pepper and Spinach

This 20-minute penne pasta recipe is paired with roasted red peppers, garlic and spinach, and served with crumbled feta cheese for a quick and simple Mediterranean-style meal.

Active Time: 20 minutes | Total Time: 20 minutes | Servings: 6 | Calories: 377 kcal

Ingredients:

- Whole-wheat penne: 12 ounces
- Garlic: 3 large cloves, diced
- Extra-virgin olive oil: ¼ cup
- Roasted red peppers: 1 jar (16 ounces), drained and chopped
- Baby spinach: 1 package (10 ounces)
- Salt: ½ teaspoon
- Ground pepper: ½ teaspoon
- Feta cheese: ¾ cup, crumbled

Directions:

1. Boil a half-filled saucepan of water, and cook pasta as instructed by the package. Drain water and return pasta to the pot.

2. In the meantime, heat oil over low-medium heat in a broad skillet. Add minced garlic and cook, frequently stirring, until fragrant.

3. Add spinach, roasted red peppers, salt and pepper and cook for about 4-5 minutes until the spinach is wilted.

4. Add pasta in the vegetable mixture. Top with crumbled feta cheese and serve.

13) Vegan Udon Soup with Noodles

This noodles recipe in Japanese-style is packed with many Asian ingredients: miso, mirin (wine) and sesame oil.

Active Time: 35-40 minutes | Total Time: 40 minutes | Servings: 4 | Calories: 325 kcal

Ingredients:

*   Udon noodles: 4 ounces

*   Canola oil: 1 tablespoon

*   Fresh garlic: 1 ½ tablespoon, minced

*   Fresh ginger: 1 tablespoon, grated

*   Serrano pepper: 1

*   Vegetable broth: 1 container (32 fluid ounce), low-sodium

*   Mirin: 1 tablespoon

*   Soy sauce: 1 tablespoon+ 1 teaspoon

*   Cremini mushrooms: 2 cups, sliced

*   Carrots: 1 cup, diced

- Baby bok choy: 2 heads, cut into 1-inch pieces
- Warm water: ½ cup
- White miso: 2 teaspoons
- Extra-firm tofu: 1 package (14 ounces), drained and cubed
- Scallions: ½ cup (4 medium), thinly sliced
- Sesame oil: 4 teaspoons, toasted, divided

Instructions:

1. Cook noodles as instructed in the package; drain water and put aside.

2. In the meantime, heat oil over low-medium heat in a broad pan. Add the ginger, garlic, and serrano; cook for about 1-2 minute, until fragrant.

3. Add mirin and broth and 1 tablespoon soy sauce and simmer. Add the carrots and mushrooms; simmer for 3-6 minutes, until the veggies are soft. Add bok choy and stir for 2 more minutes.

4. Whisk miso in warm until smooth and bring to the boil. Add tofu and cook for about 1-2 minute, until cooked through.

5. Add scallions in the broth.

6. Drizzle the soup over noodles. Sprinkle 1 teaspoon sesame oil and 1/4 teaspoon soy sauce and serve.

14) Vegan Enchilada Casserole

Prep Time: 25-30 minutes | Total Time: 1 hour | Servings: 8 | Calories: 357 kcal

Ingredients:

- Extra-virgin olive oil: 2 tablespoons
- Chopped onion: 1 cup

- Poblano peppers: ¾ cup, chopped
- Garlic: 6 cloves, minced
- Yellow squash: 1 medium, halved
- Zucchini: 1 medium, halved and sliced (1/4-inch)
- Fresh corn kernels: 1 cup
- Pico de gallo: 1 cup
- Salt: ½ teaspoon
- Pinto beans: 1 can (15 ounces), salt-free, rinsed
- Black beans: 1 can (15 ounces), salt-free, rinsed
- Corn tortillas: 8 (6 inches)
- Pepper Jack cheese: 1 ½ cups shredded
- Avocado: 1, diced
- Scallions: ½ cup
- Sour cream: ½ cup, low-fat

Instructions:

1. Set the oven to 350 F and preheat it. Heat the oil over low-moderate heat in a large skillet. Add the poblanos and garlic and cook for 4-5 minutes, frequently stirring, until softened.

2. Add cabbage, corn, zucchini, Pico de gallo and salt.

3. Cook for 5-7 minutes, occasionally stirring until the liquid decreases by half. Turn off the heat; stir in pinto beans and black beans.

4. Spray a 9/13-inch baking tray with almond oil. Spread 1/2 of the vegetable mixture onto the tray.

5. Put 4 tortillas over the mixture. Sprinkle the cheese over the tortillas evenly. Repeat the same procedure for the remaining vegetable mixture and tortillas.

6. Bake 25-30 minutes, until bubbles appear on cheese. Sprinkle with scallions and avocados, evenly.

7. Serve with sour cream.

15) Black Bean-Cauliflower "Rice" Bowl

This aromatic rice bowl of cauliflower is prepared in minutes and is a perfect dinner meal.

Active Time: 20-25 minutes | Total Time: 30 minutes | Servings: 1 | Calories: 510 kcal

Ingredients:

- Olive oil: 1 tablespoon + 2 teaspoons, divided
- Cauliflower rice: 1 cup, frozen
- Salt: ⅛ teaspoon
- Chopped onion: 2 tablespoons
- Green bell pepper: 2 tablespoons, chopped
- Chilli powder: ½ teaspoon
- Ground cumin: ½ teaspoon
- Dried oregano: ¼ teaspoon
- Canned black beans: ⅔ cup, salt-free, rinsed
- Roasted red pepper: 2 tablespoons, chopped
- Water: ¼ cup
- Lime juice: 1 tablespoon
- Cheddar cheese: ¼ cup, low-fat, shredded
- Tomato: 1 medium, chopped
- Fresh cilantro: 1 tablespoon, chopped.

Instructions:

1. Heat 1 tablespoon of oil over low-moderate heat in a skillet. Add salt and cauliflower rice; cook for 3-5 minutes, frequently stirring, until cooked through.

2. Transfer to a dish.

3. In another skillet heat the remaining 2 teaspoons of oil over low-medium heat. Add green pepper, onion, chili powder, cumin and oregano; cook for about 3-4 minutes, frequently stirring, until the veggies are softened.

4. Add roasted red pepper, beans and the water; bring to a boil. Cook 3-5 minutes, frequently stirring, until cooked and thickened. Add lime juice after turning the heat off.

5. Layer the bean mixture into a dish with the soft cauliflower rice. Top with cheese and tomato. Use cilantro for garnishing, if you like.

16) Zucchini Noodle Primavera

This recipe cut out carbohydrates by replacing the zucchini noodles with pasta. This vegan dinner is packed with colorful veggies smothered in a sweet, creamy sauce.

Active Time: 15-20 minutes | Total Time: 25-30 minutes | Servings: 4 | Calories: 313 kcal

Ingredients:

- Unsalted butter: 2 tablespoons
- All-purpose flour: 2 tablespoons (1 cup)
- Basil pesto: 3 tablespoons, refrigerated
- Extra-virgin olive oil: 1 tablespoon
- Cherry tomatoes: 2 cups, halved.
- Garlic: 4 cloves, sliced
- Salt: ¼ teaspoon
- Broccoli florets: 2 cups

- Red bell pepper: 1 cup thinly sliced

- Carrots: 1 cup, cut into matchsticks size

- Zucchini noodles: 2 packages (10 ounces), about 6 cups

- Parmesan cheese: ¼ cup, shredded

- Fresh basil: 2 tablespoons, chopped

Directions:

1. Melt the butter in a saucepan. Add flour gradually and keep on whisking until the mixture is thickened.

2. Add pesto; stir until well mixed. Turn off heat and rest aside.

3. Heat the oil over low-moderate heat in a broad skillet. Add garlic, tomatoes, and salt; cook, frequently stirring, for 3-4 minutes, until the garlic is fragrant and tomatoes turn into a paste.

4. Add bell pepper, broccoli, carrots and pesto mixture; cook for around 4-5 minutes until the broccoli is moist.

5. Add the noodles; gently shake to mix.

6. Cook for about 2-3 minutes, shaking gently until the noodles are well coated with the sauce.

7. Divide equally into 4 bowls; Serve with basil and parmesan.

17) Vegan "Pancit Bihon" with Spaghetti Squash

In this classic Filipino noodle recipe pancit bihon, shiitake mushrooms are used instead of beef, and spaghetti squash for conventional rice noodles. To make it a meal, serve with your preferred vegan main or cubed tofu.

Active Time: 20 minutes| Total Time: 1 hour| Servings: 4| Calories: 207 kcal

Ingredients:

- Spaghetti squash: 1 small, (1 3/4-2 pounds), seeds removed and halved.
- Coconut oil: 2 tablespoons
- Onion: 1 cup, chopped
- Garlic: 2 tablespoons minced
- Fresh ginger: 1 tablespoon, minced
- Shiitake mushroom caps: 2 cups sliced
- Green vegetables: 2 cups, shredded (e.g. cabbage, bok choy or kale)
- Carrot: 1 cup, shredded
- Salt: ¼ teaspoon
- Ground pepper: ¼ teaspoon
- Soy sauce: 1 tablespoon, low-sodium
- For serving: lemon wedges

Instructions:

1. Set the oven to 400 F and preheat.
2. Spread spaghetti squash, cut down in halves on a baking tray. Bake, for 35-40 minutes, until soft.
3. Once cool, remove the flesh from shells with the help of a fork.

4. Heat oil over low-medium heat in a broad skillet. Add garlic, onion and ginger, cook for 3-4 minutes until onions turn translucent. Add the mushrooms in it and cook for another 4-5 minutes, frequently stirring, until tender.

5. Add green veggies, salt and pepper and carrots; cook, stirring for 1-2 minutes until softened. Turn off the heat and stir soy sauce and spaghetti squash.

6. Garnish with lime wedges.

18) Vegan Gumbo

This vegan dinner is a classic Louisiana veggie version. It is chock-filled with tomatoes, butternut squash, poblano peppers and okra. This vegan gumbo is a fast dinner packed with flavor and spice and takes only 30 minutes active time.

Active Time: 30 minutes | Total Time: 30-35 minutes | Servings: 10 | Calories: 322 kcal

Ingredients:

- All-purpose flour: ½ cup
- Extra-virgin olive oil: ⅓ cup
- Butternut squash: 1 small, cubed into 3/4- to 1-inch
- Yellow onions: 2 cups, chopped
- Poblano peppers: 2 cups, chopped
- Celery: 1 cup, chopped
- Vegetable broth: 8 cups, low-sodium
- Whole plum tomatoes: 1 can (28 ounces), drained and crushed
- Salt: 1 ¾ teaspoon
- Okra: 3 cups, trimmed and sliced
- Zucchini: 3 cups, chopped

- Pinto beans: 2 cans (15 ounces), rinsed.
- Hot sauce: 2 tablespoons
- Red-wine vinegar: 1 tablespoon
- Ground pepper: ½ teaspoon
- Brown rice: 4 cups, cooked

Instructions:

1. In a seven-quarter pot, whisk the oil and flour.
2. Cook over low-medium heat, occasionally stirring, until the mixture is dark brown, for 10-12 minutes.
3. Add cabbage, poblanos, onions, and celery; cook for about 5-6 minutes, frequently stirring, until the veggies are well coated and moist.
4. Add water, salt and crushed tomatoes; bring to a boil. Add okra; lower heat and simmer for 5-6 minutes.
5. Add the beans and zucchini; simmer for about 4-5 minutes, until the squash is tender. Garnish with chilli sauce, vinegar and seasoning. Serve with beans.

19) Noodles with Shiitakes, Bean Sprouts and Carrots

A Sriracha hit gives this balanced vegetarian recipe a spicy and sweet edge. Modern lo mein is made from fresh lo mein noodles, available in Asian markets. You may also use dried or fresh linguine noodles. This simple dinner is prepared in just 30-35 minutes, which makes it great for weekends.

Prep Time: 35 minutes | Total Time: 40 minutes | Servings: 4 | Calories: 319 kcal

Ingredients:

- Fresh lo mein noodles: 8 ounces
- Sesame oil: 2 teaspoons, toasted
- Soy sauce: 3 tablespoons, Low-sodium

- Sriracha: 2 teaspoons
- Vegetable oil: 2 tablespoons, divided
- Minced garlic: 2 tablespoons
- Carrot: 1 large (about 1 cup), cut into half lengthwise and then cut 1/4-inch-thick half-moon shape slices
- Shiitake mushrooms: 4 ounces, stems removed and caps cut into 1/4-inch thick slices.
- Celery: 1 cup, thinly sliced
- Bean sprouts: 2 cups
- Fresh cilantro: 3 tablespoons, chopped

Instructions:

1. Bring water to boil in a half-filled pot.
2. Cook noodles as directed by box.
3. Drain the water. Move to a big bowl and sprinkle with sesame oil; rest aside.
4. In a tiny cup, mix Sriracha and soy sauce; rest aside.
5. Heat over low-medium heat a 12-inch stainless steel skillet. Add 1 tablespoon vegetable oil.
6. Add the garlic; stir-fry for about 10-12 seconds, until only fragrant. Add mushrooms, carrot and celery; stir-fry for about 1-2 minute until the celery turns bright green and the veggies have absorbed all the oil.
7. Stir in the remaining 1 tablespoon of oil. Add noodles, bean sprouts, and soy sauce; stir-fry for 1-2 minutes until the noodles are cooked through, and the veggies are crispy and tender. Add cilantro, toss and serve.

20) Spring Veggie Wraps

This veggie wrap recipe is a colorful mixture of tangy tahini-ginger-soy, both marinate the tofu and gives a spicy flavor. Go for spinach green tortillas for an extra pop.

Active Time: 25 minutes | Total: 1 hour 15 minutes | Servings: 4 | Calories: 385 kcal

Ingredients:

- 1 (14 ounces) package extra-firm tofu, drained and cut into 1/4-inch-thick planks
- Tahini sauce: ¼ cup
- Orange juice: ¼ cup + 2 tablespoons, divided
- Lime juice: 1 tablespoon
- Soy sauce, low-sodium: 1 tablespoon
- Fresh ginger: 1 tablespoon, minced
- Garlic: 1 clove, minced
- Avocado or canola oil: 2 teaspoons divided
- Salt: ¼ teaspoon, divided
- Bibb lettuce: 8 large leaves
- Carrot: 1 cup, shredded
- Radishes: 6 mediums, thinly sliced
- Scallions, thinly sliced: 2 tablespoons
- Whole-wheat tortillas: 4 8-inch warmed
- Sesame seeds: 2 tablespoons

Instructions:

1. Use a paper towel, put tofu on it and press gently to drain excess water.

2. Move the tofu to a baking tray of 9/12-inch.

3. In a medium bowl, whisk together 1/4 cup orange juice, tahini, lime juice, ginger soy sauce, and garlic.

4. Save 1/4 cup of the mixture in the refrigerator for later use as a sauce. Add 2 tablespoons orange juice in the remaining mixture. Marinate the tofu in the mixture and refrigerate for 25-30 minutes.

5. Heat 1 teaspoon oil over low-medium heat in a broad skillet.

6. Add half the marinated tofu in oil and sprinkle 1/8 teaspoon salt; toss and cook for 4-6 minutes, until golden brown.

7. Place the tofu onto a dish and keep warm. Repeat the process with remaining tofu.

8. Arrange the carrots, lettuce, radishes, and scallions down the middle of each tortilla. Add the tofu, and pour the sauce you reserved over it. Serve with a sprinkle of sesame seeds.

1.3 Delicious Vegan Dessert Recipes

Such delicious vegan and dairy-free dessert recipes (from ice cream to no-bake brownies to the yummiest cheesecake) promise to satisfy every palate, whether you are a vegan, lactose intolerant or just craving anything sweet.

1) Strawberry Coconut Cream Pie

Prep Time: 10 mins | Total Time: 10 mins | Yield: 8-10

Ingredients:

For Pie Crust:

- Medjool dates: ¾ cup (about 11), soak in warm water for 5-6 minutes, then drain the water
- Raw cashews: 3/4 cup, chopped
- Unsweetened coconut: 1/4 cup, shredded

For Pie Filling:
- Coconut cream: 1 can (14-oz), refrigerate overnight
- Maple syrup: 2 tablespoons
- Vanilla extract: 2-3 drops
- Strawberries: 1 lb., sliced
- For Pie Topping:
- Toasted coconut
- Grated dark chocolate
- Fresh mint

Instructions:
1. Crust Preparation: Add cashew bits, drained dates, and coconut in a blender and blend until the mixture can be shaped into a ball easily.
2. Layer plastic wrap on an 8-inch round-shaped cake pan.
3. Dump the cashew-date-coconut mixture into the middle of the pan and flatten it with fingertips, gently pressing the sides of the pan. Put the pan freezer to set for a few minutes.
4. Filling preparation: Take the coconut milk out of the fridge. Scoop the solid white part out and put it in a hand mixer's bowl. Add the maple syrup, vanilla and whip for around 1-2 minutes until fluffy and smooth.
5. Assembling: Take the crust out from the freezer. Pour the filling over the crust, then use a spatula to smooth out the top. Put back in the freezer for 15-20 minutes.
6. After 10 minutes take out from the freezer and top with toasted coconut, strawberries, mint. Put back in the freezer for almost an hour.
7. Remove the pie gently from the pan and wrap. Cut and serve on a serving plate.

2) Almond Apricot Tart

Ingredients:
- Pie crust: 1 9-inch
- Apricot preserves: 1/4 cup
- Slivered almonds: 3/4 cup
- Apricots: 7-9
- Sugar: 1/3 cup
- Vegan butter: 1 tablespoon, cut into small cubes

Preparation:
1. Set the oven to 450 ° F and preheat. Roll the pie crust into around 10-11 inches and spread it gently onto the pie pan, pressing firmly on both the bottom and sides. Poke the bottom of the pastry using a fork, so it does not puff up during the process of baking.
2. Bake for 10-12 minutes or until crust turn golden brown.
3. When the pastry has been removed, raise the oven temperature to 375 ° F.
4. Add the almonds in a hand blender and blend until the almonds are chopped, but not crushed to powder. Put it aside.
5. Fill a large pot with water and ice of equal parts, set aside. - Bring a casserole of half-filled water to boil and add 2 to 3 apricots in it, simmer for 20-25 seconds and move to the ice bath for immediate cooling.
6. Repeat with the remaining apricots. Then peel and slice them in half using a sharp knife, removing the pits. Put on aside.
7. Layer the apricot jam in the base of the tart. Sprinkle with chopped almonds and make a second layer of apricot halves over the almonds, cut side down. Sprinkle with some sugar and bits of butter uniformly over the tart.
8. Bake for about 50-60 minutes, until apricots are soft.
9. Cool and serve!

3) Cherry Almond Cake

Calories: 425 kcal | Serves: 6 | Cooking Time: 45 minutes

Ingredients:
- Spelt flour: 1 ¼ cup
- Almond flour: 1 ¼ cup
- Salt: 1/4 teaspoon
- Baking powder: 2 teaspoons
- Cinnamon: 1/2 teaspoons
- Coconut sugar: 1/2 cup
- Natural almond butter: 1/3 cup
- Maple syrup: 2 tablespoons
- Vanilla extract: 1/2 teaspoon (optional)
- Almond milk: 1 cup
- Cherries: 1 cup, frozen and pitted
- Slivered almonds

Preparation:
1. Set the oven to 320 °F and preheat.
2. Take a large bowl, and mix the first 6 ingredients, and stir to avoid any clumps.
3. Switch to the blender with maple syrup, almond butter, vanilla and oat milk. Blend all the ingredients.
4. Whisk the wet ingredients in a bowl. Then, fold the cherries in.
5. Move the dough to 7 inches of the lightly greased cake pan. Place a few cherries and slivered almonds on top, and gently press down.
6. Bake 45–50 minutes. Set aside to cool completely.
7. Garnish with coconut cream.

4) Skillet Strawberry S' mores

Active Time: 8-10 minutes | Cook Time: 10 minutes | Total Time: 18 minutes | Yield: 15 servings

Ingredients:
- Cast iron skillet: 8-inch
- Vegan butter: 1/2 tablespoon

- Vegan chocolate chips: 1 1/2 cups
- Vegan marshmallows: 15
- Vegan graham crackers

Instructions:

1. Put an 8-inch iron skillet into the oven's middle rack. Set the oven to 450 ° F and preheat it.
2. Once preheated, take the hot skillet out of the oven and put it on the stovetop. Coat the bottom of the pan with vegan butter. Layer the chocolate chips on the bottom of the pan, then layer the marshmallows over the chocolate chips in a way to completely cover the chocolate.
3. Put the skillet back in the oven for around 8-10 minutes, or until it on marshmallows turn light brown.
4. Serve with graham crackers right away.
5) **Peach and Cream Cheesecake**

A super easy and creamy summer cake! All vegan, gluten-free, refined sugar-free and no-bake.

Ingredients:

For the Filling:

- Cashews: 250 g, soak for 6 hours
- Maple syrup: 150 g
- Oat milk: 130 g
- Melted coconut oil: 110 g
- Lemon juice: 50 g
- Fresh peaches: 2
- Turmeric powder: 1 teaspoon
- Vanilla powder: 1/2 teaspoon
- Pinch of salt

For the Crust:

- White almonds: 200 g
- Shredded coconut: 25 g
- Pitted dates: 4

Instructions:

1. Note: The cashews can be soaked up to 24 hours before use. Only take a large tub, fill it up with the nuts and water. Bear in mind that the nuts suck up water and so leave some space for this.
2. Add the shredded coconut and almonds to your blender. Blend until you have a texture resembling flour.
3. Add the dates, and then blend again.
4. Take an 8-inch parchment paper cake pan and line with it. Press the crust into the saucepan uniformly, set aside.
5. Add the cashews with the oat milk, maple syrup, lemon juice, coconut oil, vanilla powder and salt and in the blender.
6. Fill a bowl with half the mixture. Put it aside.
7. Cut the peaches, remove the block, and add into the blender with turmeric powder.
8. Mix well and spread over the crust. Put in the freezer for 1 hour. Meanwhile, put the other bowl into your fridge with the filling.
9. Spread a second layer on the top of your peach layer and set in the freezer overnight.
10. Garnish with your choice of fresh fruits.

6) Lemon Custard

Serves: 6 | Cooking Time: 5
Ingredients:
- Soy milk, unsweetened: 4 cups
- Cornstarch: 8 tablespoons
- Sugar: 6 tablespoons
- Turmeric: 2/8 teaspoon
- 1 lemon zest
- Vanilla extract: 1 teaspoon (optional)

Preparation:
1. Whisk the cornstarch, milk, sugar and turmeric together in a saucepan until well incorporated.
2. Place the saucepan over low-moderate heat and bring it to a simmer while continually whisking. Let the starch

simmer gently for at least 1-2 minutes, frequently stirring to prevent any lumps, until desired consistency is achieved. Add the ingredients of flavoring (vanilla extract or lemon zest). If using lemon zest, make sure that only the yellow portion of the lemon is used, and not the white part under the skin.

3. Let the custard refrigerate at room temperature. Whisk occasionally to avoid skin formation on the surface. Let the pan in sit in cold water to cool down faster. Once cool serve!

7) Peanut Butter Chocolate Chip Cookie Bars

These cookies with peanut butter are my favorite treats for all time! They get a nice chocolate chip, peanut butter and a thick layer of cacao-date on top of it.

Serves: 25

Ingredients:
- Cookie Layer
- Creamy peanut butter: ½ cup + 2 tablespoons
- Melted coconut oil: ¼ cup + 1 tablespoon
- Maple syrup: ¼ cup + 1 tablespoon
- Vanilla extract: 2 teaspoons
- Heaping sea salt: ½ teaspoon
- Almond flour: 2 ½ cups
- Maca powder: 2 ½ tablespoons
- Chocolate chips: 1 cup
- Cacao Layer
- Walnuts: 1½ cups
- Cacao powder: 2 tablespoons
- Sea salt: ¼ teaspoon
- Medjool dates: 10, soft
- Water: 2 tablespoons
- For sprinkling on top: Flaky sea salt (optional)

Instructions:

1. Line parchment paper in an 8X8-inch baking pan. Stir the coconut oil, maple syrup, vanilla, peanut butter, and salt in a wide bowl, until mixed. Add maca and the almond flour and stir to blend until the mixture is thick.
2. Add the chocolate chips and fill into the pan. Put the pan in the freezer so it can firm up a little before creating the next coat.
3. Process the cacao powder, walnuts and sea salt in a food processor until the walnuts get well chopped. When the blade gets sticky, add the dates and pump to mix, add 2 tablespoons of water. Process until well combined, and then spread onto the layer of cookies. Where appropriate, sprinkle the sea salt.
4. Freeze it for 30-35 minutes (this will help them firm up and make cutting easier). Take out and slice into bars. Store the remaining bars into the fridge or freeze them. Let the bars thaw in at room temperature for around 13-15 minutes.

8) Chocolate Avocado Pudding Pops

Prep time: 9 hours 5 minutes | Total time: 9 hours 5 mins | Serves: 10 pops

This recipe of chocolate pudding is a great summer dessert! It is completely vegetarian because almond butter and avocado make the base smooth and creamy.

Ingredients:
- Ripe avocados: 2 mediums
- Chocolate chips: ¼ cup, melted
- Cocoa powder: 3 tablespoons
- Maple syrup: 3 tablespoons
- Almond butter: 3 tablespoons
- Vanilla extract: 1 teaspoon
- Almond milk Vanilla: 2 cups
- Sea salt: ¼ teaspoon

Topping:
- Chocolate chips: ½ cup

- Coconut oil: + ½ teaspoon
- Crushed nuts: pistachios or almonds

Instructions:

1. Add the avocados with the almond milk, maple syrup, cocoa powder, almond butter, cinnamon, sea salt and melted chocolate chips into a blender. Mix until smooth. Pour in the ice pop moulds and place in the freeze overnight, or for 9 hours or more.
2. Before removing, let the pops settle for a couple of minutes at room temperature and loose enough to pull out.
3. Additional topping: Mix the coconut oil and melted chocolate chips and drizzle on the pops, also sprinkle the nuts.
4. Instead, this can be eaten as pudding. Scoop into a blender or individual bowls after you combine the mixture, and chill in the refrigerator for at least 2-4 hours.

9) Best Vegan Ice Cream

Active Time: 20-25 minutes | Total time: 30 minutes | Serves: 4
This simple, milk-free ice cream is so delightful and rich! In this recipe, the tahini has no strong flavor; it just gives the base of coconut milk an extra-creamy texture.

Ingredients:

- Full-fat coconut milk: 1 can (14-ounce)
- Maple syrup: ⅓ cup
- Tahini: ¼ cup
- Toppings:
- Tart cherries
- Sesame seeds
- Chocolate

Instructions:

1. Refrigerate your Ice Cream Attachment frame for minimum 12 hours, ideally overnight.

2. Mix the maple syrup, tahini and coconut milk together in a wide cup. (If the coconut milk is chunky, you can put the ingredients together in a blender).
3. Pour the mixture into the ice cream machine, and churn for about 20 minutes until warm. Scoop out and have fun!
4. Freeze it for 1-2 hours, if you like thick texture.

Note:
If you have your ice cream stored in the refrigerator for more than 24 hours, it can harden. Set aside at room temperature to soften before scooping for 20 minutes.

10) Blackberry and White Chocolate Tart

Ingredients:
Crust:
- Oat flour: 1 cup
- Almond milk: 1 cup
- Maple syrup: 2-3 tablespoons (optional)
- Coconut oil: 1/4 cup
- Pinch of salt

For Filling:
- Cashews: 3/4 cup, soaked for 4-5 hours
- Fresh blackberries: 1 cup
- White chocolate (vegan): 200g
- Full-fat coconut milk: 2 cans
- Maple syrup: 1/4 cup
- Super color powder: 1/4 teaspoon
- Agar powder: 1 teaspoon

For Garnishing:
- Delaware grapes
- Fresh blackberries

Instructions:
Crust:

1. Set your oven at 180 Celsius. Oil an 8 inches tart plate. Set aside. Mix the crust ingredients into a food processor and mix well.
2. You must get a sticky mixture that can quickly be molded. Press tightly to the base and up the walls of the tart pan. Bake it for 25 mins until the crust becomes golden brown.
3. Move to a rack and let it cool while you prepare the filling.

Filling:
1. Place the saucepan over a low-medium heat and add the blackberries with 2 tablespoons of water. As it starts boiling mash the blackberries. Strain it and let them cool down. In a saucepan, add white chocolate and melt it then add coconut cream, and put at low heat. Add the maple syrup, agar-agar, and super color powder and make the mixture moist.
2. Stir it repeatedly, cook until the agar dissolves. Put the soaked cashew nuts, blackberry mixture, and the white chocolate-coconut cream into a food processor and blend.
3. Continue until smooth.
4. Fill the crust with this mixture. Place the tart overnight in the refrigerator to set. Garnish, and have fun!

11) Coconut Mango Panna Cotta

Makes 4-6 depending Panna Cottas
Ingredients:
For the Panna Cotta:
- Coconut milk, unsweetened: 3 cups
- Maple syrup: 4 tablespoons
- Agar powder: 1 teaspoon
- Vanilla extract: ½ teaspoon

For the Jelly:
- Mango purée: 1 cup
- Maple syrup: 1 tablespoon (optional)

- Agar powder: ½ teaspoon
- For garnishing:
- Toasted coconut chips

Directions:

For the Panna Cotta:

1. Whisk all the ingredients together in a normal-sized pan over low-medium heat.
2. Boil the mixture and turn off the burner instantly. In 4-6 glasses or ramekins, equally, pour the mixture.
3. Let it refrigerate for 3-4 hours, until set.

For the Jelly:

1. In a medium-sized saucepan, over low-medium heat, whisk all the ingredients and bring it to boil.
2. Turn off the heat and allow for several minutes to cool down before pouring over. Transfer the panna cotta to the refrigerator for one hour to set the mango.
3. Before serving, toss the coconut chips on the top.

12) Frozen Yogurt Bars

An amazing homemade frozen Greek yoghurt bars with berries, or variations of your favorite fruit. Vegetarian and gluten-free, ideal for breakfast, a balanced meal!

Active Time: 10-15 minutes | Cook Time: 3 minutes | Freezing time: 4 hours | Total Time: 15 minutes | Servings: 10 people | Calories: 64kcal

Ingredients:

- Greek-style yogurt (Vegan): 2 cups
- Blueberries: 5 oz
- Fresh blackberries: 2 oz
- Vanilla extract: 1 teaspoon
- Juice of ½ lemon
- Maple syrup: 4 tablespoons

Instructions:

1. In a wide pan, add the blueberries and the lemon juice and bring it to a boil. Cook well until the blueberries have mixed up and let it cool.

2. Mix the Greek yogurt, maple syrup and vanilla in a medium dish. When cooled, add in blueberry sauce.
3. Layer a parchment paper in a baking dish and pour the yogurt mix in it.
4. Toss with some fresh blackberries, and freeze until solid for 4 to 5 hours. Slice them into bars of 2-3 inches, and enjoy.

13) Vegan Chocolate Pudding Recipe

Active time: 10-15 minutes | Cook time: 10 minutes | Chilling time: 4 hours | Yield: 4 to 8 servings

Ingredients:
- Full-fat coconut milk: 1 (15-ounce) can
- Dark chocolate (60-70%): 10 ounces, finely chopped
- Vanilla extract: 1 tablespoon, (optional)

For Garnishing:
- Shaved chocolate
- Whipped coconut cream
- Berries or other fresh fruit

Instructions:
1. Shake the coconut milk's can, before opening and pour into a small saucepan and warm it. Heat up coconut milk over low heat to a simmer. Stir in regularly to prevent scorching. Warm-up for a few minutes, until the liquid nearly boils. Remove it from heat immediately.
2. Add the chocolate:
3. Add 1/3 of the chopped chocolate in the hot coconut milk. Mix it gently until the chocolate has melted fully, and the paste is smooth. Continue in two different combinations, with the remaining chocolate. Whisk and add in the vanilla extract.
4. Take out the mixture into ramekins, glasses or jars. Wrap the plastic foil and place in the refrigerate for 4 hours.
5. To serve: Remove about 25 minutes before from the refrigerator. Top with your favorite toppings or simply serve with a spoon.

14) Vegan Mango Mousse

A Mousse, veggie-free, sugar-friendly and nice to taste! In this recipe, there is no gelatin or agar-agar, and it almost finished without additional sweetness.

Active Time: 12-15 minutes | Total Time: 1 hour | Servings: 4 people | Calories: 290 kcal

Ingredients:
- Mangoes: 3
- Coconut cream: 1 ½ cup
- Agave syrup: 3 tablespoons
- Powdered sugar: 2 tablespoons

Instructions:
1. Peel and slice the mangoes. Mash the slices to make a thick puree. Place the coconut cream in a large cup, and whisk the mango puree gently until it is smooth.
2. Add 3 tbsps of agave or sugar.
3. Season the Mousse with chocolate or shavings of fresh fruit.
4. This is it! Cool for 2-3 hours, and serve chilled!

15) Black and White Bombs

Ingredients:
- Slivered almonds: 2 cups
- Coconut oil: 1 cup
- Powdered sweetener: 1 - 2 tablespoon
- Vanilla extract: 2 teaspoons
- Orange zest: 1 teaspoon
- A pinch of kosher salt

Instructions:
1. Fill a small 12 cups muffin tray with small liners.
2. In a food processor, process the almonds oil, sweetener, zest and salt to a smooth mixture. Put the half mixture into a small bowl and add in powdered cocoa and whisk it.

3. Fill half of the muffin tray with the cocoa mixture and another half with vanilla. (You can have two colored cookies)
4. Repeat this process with the remaining mixture. Tap the tray on the table to prevent bubbles.
5. Freeze for about 25-30 minutes, until firm. Remove the liners if you want.
6. Put it in the fridge for max 4-5 days in an airtight jar.

16) Pineapple, Banana, Strawberry Skewers with Salted Chocolate Drizzle

Cook Time: 10 minutes| Prep Time: 15 minutes| Servings: 4 servings

Ingredients:
- Pineapple: 2 cups, cut into 1 1/2 -inch cubes
- Strawberries: 8
- Bananas: 2, sliced into 1 1/2-inch thick circles
- Coconut oil: 2 teaspoons
- Dark chocolate chips: 1/3 cup
- Coconut oil: 2 teaspoons
- Sea salt: 1/2 tsp
- Unsweetened coconut: 1/2 cup, toasted and shredded

Directions:
1. Use your skewers, to thread the pineapple pieces, bananas, and strawberries. Must soak in the water, when you use wooden skewers.
2. Heat the grill to low flame, put the fruits and brush with almond oil to avoid sticking.
3. Cook the skewers of fruits on the hot grill, for 2-3 minutes each side.
4. Turn off the grill and put the fruits on a tray. In a double boiler, make the chocolate dressing by heating up the coconut oil, choc chips and sea salt.
5. Keep swirling the chocolate till it is creamy, and then drizzle all over the fruits.
6. When you are not drizzling it on top, serve extra dipping with it.
7. Sprinkle with toasted chopped coconut, and voila!

17) Mint Chocolate Chip Ice Cream

Prep Time: 15-10 minutes | Total Time: 4 hours, 15 minutes
Ingredients:
- Avocados: 2, peeled and pitted
- Full-fat coconut milk: 1 14 oz can
- Cashews: 1 cup
- Coconut oil: 1 tablespoon
- Medjool dates: 10
- Cacao nibs: 1/4 cup
- Mint leaves: 3/4 cup
- Vanilla extract: 1 tsp
- Sea salt: 1/4 tsp
- Liquid chlorophyll: 1 tablespoon (for color, optional)
- Chocolate Sauce Topping:
- Dark chocolate chips: 1/3 cup
- Coconut oil: 1 teaspoon

Directions:

1. For 2-3 hours, put the coconut milk in the freezer or overnight in the refrigerator.
2. In warm water, soak the cashews for at least 2 hours, and the dates for 15 mins.
3. Once you have cooled the coconut milk, open the can and take out the tough cream from the top and put it into your food processor. You can reserve the liquid, make smoothies by using it.
4. Drain the dates and cashews, and put them with all ingredients to the blender except the cacao nibs. While it is blending, use it to move the ingredients towards the blade when your blender comes with a plunger.
5. Or just keep stopping, scrape down the sides and blend. It will take approximately 5 mins.
6. Into a loaf pan lined with parchment, pour the ice cream, using a silicone spatula, make sure you get everything out of the blender.
7. Blend the cacao nibs until well blended.
8. Use plastic foil to cover the pan and freeze for 4-5 hours or until you are ready to eat.
9. Make homemade melted chocolate in a double boiler, by melting chocolate chips and spoon in coconut oil until silky; drizzle them directly over ice cream.

18) Vegan Blueberry Muffins

Active Time: 15-20 Minutes | Total Time: 40-45 Minutes | Serves: 12

Ingredients:

- Cooking spray
- All-purpose flour: 2 cups
- Baking powder: 2 teaspoons
- Kosher salt: ½ teaspoon
- Brown sugar: ⅔ cup
- Soy milk yogurt: ½ cup
- Almond milk, unsweetened: ⅓ cup

- Vegetable oil: ⅓ cup
- Applesauce, unsweetened: ¼ cup
- Vanilla extract: 1 teaspoon
- Blueberries: 2 cups
- Turbinado sugar: 2 tablespoons

Instructions:

1. Set your oven at 350°F. Fill a 12-muffin baking tray with paper liners, and brush with cooking spray.
2. In a wide bowl, whisk together the baking powder, flour and salt. In another medium bowl, whisk the yogurt, vanilla, almond milk, brown sugar, butter and applesauce together.
3. With a spatula, gently mix the dry and wet mixture. Shortly before the batter gets thoroughly combined, mix in the blueberries. Equally, divide the batter among the muffin tray. Sprinkle the turbinado sugar on the muffin tops — Bake for 20-24 mins and test by inserting a knife in the center until it comes out clean. Let the tray cool for a couple of minutes, then remove and place on a rack.

19) Peanut Butter Cups

Makes: 12

Ingredients:

Vegan chocolate chips: 1 bag (approximately 1 1/2 cups)
Peanut butter: 1/4 cup

Directions:

1. Place a paper liner in a muffin tray or use a silicone muffin tray
2. Then melt the chocolate chips in a boiler until its smooth. On the bottom of the muffin liners, put 1 tablespoon of melted chocolate and spread it evenly with a spatula. Let it sit in the fridge for 10-15 minutes.
3. Then put 1 tablespoon of peanut butter on top of the chocolate which is hardened. Do not spread this out with your finger as it settles down and mostly remains in the middle. Refrigerate for 10 minutes.

4. When your chocolate has become sludger, just put it back in the double boiler to re-melt it quickly. Now take 1 or 2 more teaspoons of melted chocolate and bring it over the peanut butter. The peanut butter is not going to be super hard, but it is going to hold up for the remaining process.
5. Using your knife, you could even spread the melted chocolate a little in the sides to make sure it runs down to cover the peanut. It will not happen, particularly if the peanut butter portion is not refrigerated.
6. If you want, smooth the top of the cups, but they might just settle comfortably on their own. So, cool it down for at least 15-20 minutes before serving. If you want softer cups, place them in the refrigerator in an airtight jar or at room temperature.

20) Cocoa Silken Pudding

Active Time: 5 Minutes | Total Time: 5-10 Minutes | Serves: 1
Ingredients:
- Silken tofu: 1 block (19 oz)
- Raw cacao powder: ¼ cup
- Maple syrup: 3 - 4 tablespoon
- Almond milk: 1 tablespoon
- Sea salt: a pinch

Instructions:
1. Blend all the ingredients in a hand blender until smooth and creamy.
2. When you use cocoa powder, it tastes very bitter, so just put 1 tbsp of maple syrup or honey to make it taste sweeter.
3. For the extra sweet and salty combination, sprinkle a pinch of sea salt over the top, when serving the pudding.

Part 2: 7 Day Sample Meal Plans

This part covers sample meal plans covering the whole week of vegan meals to help you begin with the vegan diet and improving your strength and endurance.

Chapter 2: Sample Meal Plans to increase Strength and Endurance

Vegans may be at elevated risk for deficiencies of other nutrients. A well-planned vegan diet that contains fortified nutrient-rich foods will help to provide a sufficient level of nutrients. Here are 2 sample meal plans mentioned below for vegan athletes.

Meal plan 1 is a high-carb, low-fat plan with a 50% carb, 25% fat and 25% protein macronutrient ratios that will help you boost your strength.

Meal plan 2 is a low-carb, high-fat plan with a 30% carb, 45% fat and 25% protein macronutrient ratios, perfect for increasing stamina.

Both meal plans contain a significant amount of protein that is 25% of the total calories.

Whether you are eating a diet higher or lower in carbs depends on:

- Your skin
- The goals
- Your genetic makeup
- The sport and level of operation

No one can tell how to eat, so you are not expected to adjust what to eat based on what works for someone. It may take some research to find it out. However, most people do better with a moderate intake of about 50% carbs, with the majority of their calories coming from proteins and fats.

2.1 Vegan Sample Meal Plan for Increasing Strength

A high-carb and low-fat meal plan to give your strength a boost!

Monday

- Breakfast: Tofu scramble and a plant-milk chai latte.

- Snacks: Fruit and nut butter

- Lunch: Tofu Tacos and vegetarian kale Caesar salad.

- Dinner: Roasted veggie brown rice bowl.

Tuesday

- Breakfast: Overnight oats with fruits on the bottom, fortified plant milk, chia seeds and nuts.

- Snacks: Guacamole and crackers

- Lunch: Edamame hummus wraps.

- Dinner: Thai peanut curry noodles.

Wednesday

- Breakfast: A glass of mango and spinach smoothie and an easy baked oatmeal muffin.

- Snacks: Roasted Chickpeas

- Lunch: Stuffed potatoes with salsa and beans.

- Dinner: Black bean cauliflower rice bowl.

Thursday

- Breakfast: Whole-grain toast with banana, hazelnut butter and a fortified plant yogurt.

- Snacks: Edamame with sea salt

- Lunch: Cabbage lentil soup.

- Dinner: Eggplant Lasagna.

Friday

- Breakfast: Chocolate chip oatmeal cookie pancakes and a cappuccino made with fortified plant milk.

- Snacks: Hummus and Veggies.

- Lunch: Spring veggie wraps.

- Dinner: Vegan black bean burgers.

Saturday

- Breakfast: Avocado-Tofu toast and a glass of simple strawberry smoothie.

- Snacks: Rice cakes and avocado.

- Lunch: Roasted red pepper and ginger soup with whole-grain toast and hummus.

- Dinner: Roasted veggie brown rice bowl.

Sunday

- Breakfast: Sweet potato bowl and a glass of fortified orange juice.

- Snacks: Fruit and nut bars

- Lunch: Vegetarian lettuce wraps with a side of sautéed mustard greens.

- Dinner: Zucchini noodles primavera.

Remember to vary your carbs and protein sources during the day, as each provides various vitamins and minerals which are important for good health.

2.2 Vegan Sample Meal Plan for Increasing Endurance

A low-carb and high-fat meal plan to boost your stamina!

Monday

- Breakfast: Jelly chia pudding with peanut butter with a glass of strawberry smoothie.
- Snacks: Strawberry rolls with a bowl of oatmeal.
- Lunch: Black bean chili with sweet potato and avocado salad.
- Dinner: Soybeans hummus wraps.

Tuesday

- Breakfast: Mushroom bacon toast with hummus and a glass of spinach, mango and banana Juice.
- Snacks: 2 nutty fruit bars.
- Lunch: Thai curry noodles with peanuts.
- Dinner: Vegan soup with noodles.

Wednesday

- Breakfast: A glass of carrot mango, spinach smoothie with burritos filled with tofu.
- Snacks: A banana with 1 or 2 tablespoons of raw cashew butter.
- Lunch: Stuffed potatoes with salsa beans and spring vegetable salad.
- Dinner: Vegetarian lettuce wraps.

Thursday

- Breakfast: Tater tot waffles and a grapefruit mango smoothie.

- Snacks: Cocoa strawberry balls with vegan protein pancakes.
- Lunch: Purple artichoke pizza with asparagus.
- Dinner: Black bean-cauliflower rice bowl.

Friday

- Breakfast: Black bean and sweet potato burritos with a glass of carrot, spinach and ginger juice.
- Snacks: A bowl of berries with some yogurt and rice cakes with avocado.
- Lunch: Mexican salad with tortilla croutons.
- Dinner: Zucchini noodle primavera.

Saturday

- Breakfast: A glass of gazpacho delight with chocolate chip and oatmeal pancakes.

Snacks: hummus with veggies, 1 orange or raw seeds and nuts.

- Lunch: Spinach and apple salad.
- Dinner: Penne pasta with spinach and roasted red pepper.

Sunday

- Breakfast: Cinnamon butter fig toasts with mango carrot and banana basil smoothie.
- Snacks: salsa with tortilla chips, 1 green apple and 2 tablespoons of raw almond butter
- Lunch: Tomato and rice soup with chickpeas.
- Dinner: Noodles with shiitakes, bean sprouts and carrots.

Conclusion

Athletes following a vegan diet or contemplating a vegan diet should pay careful attention to what they are consuming. Be sure to select nutrient-dense foods from the 100 delicious recipes listed above that include carbohydrate, protein and fat with enough nutrition, plus the minerals and vitamins needed to help oxygen delivery, recovery and immunity. Choose nutritious meals and snacks to fuel you without any gastrointestinal discomfort, before and after exercise. After your workouts, your food choices will help recovery too. It is crucial for all athletes, but particularly for vegans, to choose the right meals/snacks after practice.

If you are f1ollowing a vegan diet, check the sample meal plans and make sure you are selecting the right meals. If you need help, ask a sports dietitian for advice.